RHEUMATOID ARTHRITIS RELIEF DIET

ANTI-INFLAMMATORY DIET PLAN

Dr. PRITHVI INDIRAKUMAR

Dr. PRITHVI INDIRAKUMAR MANGUDIMARUTHAN

6/50, Marulayampalayam, Salem, Tamilnadu, INDIA 637 501

Email us: drprithvidental@gmail.com

This book, "RHEUMATOID ARTHRITIS RELIEF DIET: ANTI-INFLAMMATORY DIET PLAN " is intended for informational purposes only and should not be considered as professional medical advice.

RHEUMATOID ARTHRITIS RELIEF DIET: ANTI-INFLAMMATORY DIET PLAN

Hardcopy, Paperback, 1st edition ISBN-13: **9798870299983**

Published on 29th November 2023

Published by Dr.PRITHVIINDIRAKUMAR MANGUDIMARUTHAN

Dedicated to

My Dear Father
MANGUDI MARUTHAN

My Dear Mother
RADHA MANGUDIMARUTHAN

My Dear Brother
LAKSMAN JAYASANKAR

Preface

In the world of human health, there exists an ongoing quest to empower individuals, alleviate suffering, and improve the quality of life. Amidst this noble pursuit, the prevalence of Rheumatoid Arthritis (RA) stands as a formidable challenge, affecting countless lives and posing intricate hurdles to those affected.

The journey into crafting this book began with a profound understanding of the burdens faced by individuals battling RA. The prevalence of this condition, impacting lives with its persistent and often debilitating symptoms, spurred the realization of a pressing need for comprehensive guidance and support.

My aspiration to contribute meaningfully to society sparked the genesis of this book. It is an offering aimed at enhancing the lives of those enduring the trials of Rheumatoid Arthritis. The aim is to provide a beacon of guidance, an arsenal of knowledge, and a pathway towards better management and understanding of this condition.

This book is not solely an assembly of words; it is an embodiment of compassion, a dedication to disseminate valuable insights, and a commitment to contributing to a healthier, more informed society. It's a pledge to extend a helping hand to those navigating the complexities of Rheumatoid Arthritis.

My hope is that within these pages, readers will find not just information, but empowerment; not just guidance, but solace; and not just strategies, but a sense of control. May this book serve as a valuable resource, a companion in the pursuit of managing and understanding Rheumatoid Arthritis.

Together, let us embark on a journey for a better tomorrow for all those impacted by Rheumatoid Arthritis.

Who is this Book for?

This book is crafted for individuals impacted by Rheumatoid Arthritis, whether newly diagnosed, managing the condition for years, or supporting a loved one navigating this complex journey. Specifically, it caters to:

1. **Those Diagnosed with Rheumatoid Arthritis:** Whether in the early stages or long-term management, this book offers insights to enhance understanding and manage the condition proactively.
2. **Family Members and Caregivers:** For those supporting individuals living with Rheumatoid Arthritis, providing a better grasp of the condition and offering strategies for comprehensive support.
3. **Individuals Seeking General Understanding:** Intended for anyone desiring a broader comprehension of Rheumatoid Arthritis, including those interested in autoimmune conditions, fostering empathy, or gaining insights into the experiences of individuals living with RA, to enhance their overall awareness and knowledge base.
4. **Community Support Groups and Organizations:** Providing valuable information to further educate and support their members in navigating the challenges posed by Rheumatoid Arthritis.
5. **Those Seeking Preventative Measures:** Offering insights into a diet that may help reduce the risk or severity of Rheumatoid Arthritis symptoms for those at risk or in the early stages.

This book aims to cater to a diverse audience seeking knowledge, guidance, and practical strategies to manage and understand Rheumatoid Arthritis. It serves as a companion for those seeking to take an informed and proactive approach towards their health and well-being in the face of this challenging condition.

Disclaimer

The information presented in this book is for informational purposes only. It is not intended as a substitute for professional medical advice, diagnosis, or treatment. Readers are encouraged to seek the guidance of qualified healthcare professionals for specific medical advice or treatment tailored to their individual circumstances.

The content provided in this book is based on general knowledge and research available. Given the dynamic nature of medical research and individual variations in health conditions, the information might not be universally applicable. Readers are advised to consider their unique health status, consult with healthcare providers, and verify the suitability of any suggestions or recommendations before implementation.

While every effort has been made to ensure the accuracy and relevance of the information provided, the author, contributors, and publishers do not assume responsibility for any errors, omissions, or adverse outcomes resulting from the use of the information presented in this book. Additionally, any products, medications or treatments (if any) mentioned in this book does not imply endorsement or guarantee of its effectiveness.

Readers are encouraged to use their discretion and judgment in applying the information from this book to their individual circumstances. The author, contributors, and publishers are not liable for any direct or indirect consequences resulting from the use or misuse of the information presented in this book.

Embrace Relief with the Rheumatoid Arthritis Diet

Discover Your Path to Lasting Relief

Welcome to the gateway of your journey toward renewed vitality and comfort! If you've landed here, you're seeking something more than just a book — you're seeking a solution. This is not just a collection of dietary suggestions; it's a transformative roadmap crafted to alleviate the grip of rheumatoid arthritis (RA) on your life.

Your Key to Freedom

Living with Rheumatoid Arthritis (hereafter will be abbreviated as RA) can feel like navigating a maze of discomfort, but fear not; you hold the key to unlock relief. This book isn't just about adapting what's on your plate; it's about reclaiming your life, one delicious meal at a time. It's a comprehensive guide, meticulously crafted to empower you with the knowledge and tools needed to alleviate pain and inflammation.

A Personalized Approach

Understanding that each individual's journey with RA is unique, this book offers a tailored approach. You'll find a diverse range of strategies, from nutritional insights and meal plans to lifestyle adjustments, all designed to suit your specific needs and preferences.

Empowerment Through Knowledge

In these pages, you'll delve into the science behind the foods you consume, discovering their impact on inflammation and joint health. You'll gain the confidence to make informed choices, understanding how each bite can contribute to your well-being.

Your Support System

Consider this book your trusted companion on this transformative expedition. It's not just about information; it's about walking alongside you as you navigate the twists and turns, offering guidance, encouragement, and unwavering support.

Take the First Step

By turning these pages, you're not just seeking information; you're embracing change. You're taking the first step toward a life where RA doesn't dictate your every move, where pain doesn't overshadow your joy.

The Journey Begins Now

So, embark on this journey with us. Together, let's explore, learn, and thrive. Relief from rheumatoid arthritis is not a distant dream; it's a tangible reality waiting for you within these chapters.

In this book, you'll find the tools, encouragement, and reassurance you seek. Turn the page, and let's walk this path together toward the relief you deserve!

touch, and visibly swollen due to the accumulation of excess fluid. This inflammation is a result of the immune system attacking the synovium, the lining of the joints, leading to its thickening and the production of excess synovial fluid.

Systemic Impact

The impacts of RA extend beyond the joints. The systemic nature of this condition can affect various organs, leading to complications such as cardiovascular issues, lung problems, and an increased risk of osteoporosis. Additionally, fatigue, depression, and overall reduced quality of life are common among individuals with RA.

Impact on Daily Life

The impact of rheumatoid arthritis extends beyond physical symptoms, affecting various aspects of an individual's life. The chronic pain and stiffness associated with RA can significantly limit mobility, making routine tasks like walking, grasping objects, or even getting dressed challenging in the later stages of this condition.

Simple actions like opening jars, buttoning shirts, or holding utensils can become arduous tasks. Additionally, the fatigue commonly associated with RA can be overwhelming, further hampering one's ability to engage in daily activities with energy and enthusiasm.

Moreover, the unpredictability of RA symptoms often leads to emotional distress and mental fatigue. The uncertainty of symptom flare-ups and their varying intensities can cause anxiety and stress, impacting emotional well-being and overall quality of life.

Understanding these manifestations of RA is crucial in developing effective strategies to manage and mitigate its effects on daily life.

1.2 Causes and Triggers

Rheumatoid arthritis (RA) is a complex autoimmune disorder characterized by chronic inflammation in the joints. The causes and triggers of RA encompass a blend of genetic predisposition and environmental influences.

Genetic Factors

Family History

A substantial body of evidence suggests a hereditary link to RA. Individuals with a family history of RA are at an increased risk of developing the condition. Studies indicate that having a first-degree relative such as Father, Mother or even Siblings with RA elevates the likelihood of its onset. Genetic variations inherited from parents may contribute significantly to the susceptibility to RA.

Genetic Predisposition

Certain genetic markers have been identified, revealing a predisposition to RA. The human leukocyte antigen (HLA) gene complex, particularly the HLA-DRB1 gene, has been strongly associated with RA development. Variations in this gene affect the immune system's ability to differentiate between self and foreign substances, potentially triggering an autoimmune response against healthy joint tissues.

Environmental Triggers

Diet and Lifestyle

The interplay between diet, lifestyle, and RA onset is a subject of growing interest. Certain dietary components, such as processed foods high in sugars and unhealthy fats, have been linked to increased inflammation in the body. Moreover, lifestyle factors like smoking and obesity have been identified as potential triggers, exacerbating the risk and severity of RA.

Stress and Other Factors

Stress, often underestimated, can significantly impact the immune system and inflammatory responses in the body. Chronic stress may trigger or exacerbate RA symptoms by influencing the release of stress hormones, which in turn can affect immune function. Additionally, exposure to certain infections or environmental factors, such as pollution or toxins, could potentially act as triggers for RA in susceptible individuals.

Age & Gender

Women are more commonly affected by RA than men due to decreased hormonal levels after menopause. RA can occur at any age, but most commonly seen between ages of 40 & 60.

Obesity

Obesity is associated with chronic low-grade inflammation, adipose tissue produces cytokines, which can promote inflammation & contributes to RA.

Coexisting Conditions

Individuals with other autoimmune disorders such as lupus or psoriasis, have higher risk of RA. Poor oral health specifically periodontal (gum) disease has increased risk of RA.

While genetic predisposition lays the groundwork for susceptibility, environmental factors play a crucial role in triggering the onset or exacerbation of RA symptoms. The intricate interplay between genetic and environmental factors in the development of RA highlights the importance of personalized approaches to treatment and lifestyle modifications.

1.3 Development of Rheumatoid Arthritis

Autoimmune Origin of Rheumatoid Arthritis

Rheumatoid Arthritis (RA) is fundamentally an autoimmune disease characterized by the immune system mistakenly attacking the body's tissues, particularly the synovium in joints. The immune system, usually responsible for defending against harmful pathogens, malfunctions and begins assaulting healthy tissues.

Immune System Dysfunction: RA's primary mechanism involves an immune system dysfunction where the body's defense mechanisms, particularly T cells, become hyperactive. These cells invade the synovium, causing inflammation and damage.

Role of Autoantibodies: Autoantibodies like rheumatoid factor (RF) and anti-citrullinated protein antibodies (ACPAs) play a pivotal role in RA's pathogenesis. They contribute to the immune system's attack on healthy joint tissues, exacerbating inflammation and joint degradation.

Inflammatory Processes in RA

Synovial Inflammation: The synovial membrane becomes inflamed, resulting in the proliferation of synovial cells and the formation of pannus, a destructive tissue that damages joints. This ongoing inflammation leads to pain, stiffness, and joint deformity.

Cytokine and Chemokine Activity: Pro-inflammatory molecules like tumor necrosis factor (TNF), interleukins (IL-1, IL-6), and chemokines drive the inflammatory cascade in RA. They promote immune cell activation and further inflammation, contributing to joint damage.

Genetic and Environmental Factors

Genetic Predisposition: Certain genes, notably HLA-DRB1, contribute to an increased susceptibility to RA. Individuals with specific genetic variations are more prone to developing the disease.

Environmental Triggers: Environmental factors like smoking, infections, and exposure to toxins can trigger or aggravate RA in genetically predisposed individuals. These factors can provoke the immune system, escalating the autoimmune response.

Role of Cellular Immunity

T Lymphocytes: CD4+ T cells, a type of T lymphocyte, play a critical role in RA's pathogenesis by activating the immune response against healthy tissues. Their aberrant activation leads to persistent inflammation in the joints.

Macrophages and Synovial Inflammation: Macrophages present in the synovium release inflammatory mediators, perpetuating joint inflammation and tissue damage. Their activity contributes significantly to the destructive nature of RA.

Joint Destruction and Systemic Impact

Cartilage and Bone Erosion: Enzymes released during the inflammatory process lead to the erosion of cartilage and bone within the joints. This erosion results in joint deformities, pain, and loss of function.

Systemic Effects: RA is not confined to joint damage; it has systemic effects, impacting organs and tissues beyond joints due to chronic inflammation. This chronic inflammation can affect the cardiovascular system, lungs, and other organs, leading to various complications.

Each aspect of RA's development plays a crucial role in understanding the disease's complexity, aiding in the development of strategies for management and relief through dietary and lifestyle interventions.

1.4 Diagnosis and Medical Treatments

Diagnostic Procedures

Blood Tests and Imaging

Blood tests and imaging techniques are vital in diagnosing rheumatoid arthritis (RA). Physicians rely on several blood tests to detect specific antibodies and markers indicative of RA. The **Rheumatoid factor (RF)** test identifies antibodies present in about 80% of individuals with RA, although its absence doesn't rule out the condition. Another crucial test is the **Anti-Cyclic Citrullinated Peptide (anti-CCP) antibody test**, often more sensitive in early detection.

Moreover, the **erythrocyte sedimentation rate (ESR) and C-reactive protein (CRP) tests** measure inflammation levels in the body. While elevation in these markers isn't exclusive to RA, their presence alongside other symptoms aids in diagnosis. These blood tests complement clinical assessments, forming a comprehensive diagnostic approach.

Imaging techniques like **X-rays, Ultrasounds, and MRIs** contribute significantly to RA diagnosis. X-rays reveal joint damage, including erosions and cartilage loss. Ultrasounds provide real-time images of inflamed joints and detect synovial inflammation. MRIs offer detailed views of affected tissues and are particularly useful in early disease detection when X-rays might appear normal.

Criteria for Diagnosis

The American College of Rheumatology (ACR) and the European League Against Rheumatism (EULAR) jointly established classification criteria for RA diagnosis. These criteria aid in standardizing diagnosis and ensure prompt initiation of treatment. The criteria include joint involvement, symptom duration, serologic markers, and acute-phase reactants. A patient meeting these criteria is more likely to receive a confirmed RA diagnosis.

Conventional Treatments

Medications and Therapies

Medical treatments for RA aim to alleviate symptoms, halt disease progression, and improve quality of life. Nonsteroidal anti-inflammatory drugs **(NSAIDs)** and **Corticosteroids** are commonly prescribed to manage pain and inflammation. Disease-modifying antirheumatic drugs **(DMARDs)** such as methotrexate, hydroxychloroquine, and sulfasalazine are pivotal in suppressing the immune system and slowing joint damage.

Biologic response modifiers (Biologics) or **Immunomodulators** are another class of medications used when conventional DMARDs prove ineffective. These drugs target specific components of the immune system involved in RA, offering better disease control for some patients.

Physical therapy helps maintain joint mobility and strength, while occupational therapy assists in adapting daily activities to reduce joint stress. Assistive devices and splints may also alleviate discomfort and improve function.

Surgery Options

Joint replacement surgery, particularly for knees and hips, is a viable option for severe joint damage. **Synovectomy**, involving the removal of the inflamed synovial tissue, done to alleviate pain and prevent further joint destruction. In extreme cases, joint fusion or **Joint reconstruction surgeries** are considered to restore function and reduce pain.

Accurate diagnosis through blood tests, imaging, and adherence to standardized criteria enables timely initiation of appropriate treatments. Conventional treatments like medications, therapies, and, when necessary, surgical interventions aim to mitigate symptoms and slow disease progression, significantly improving the quality of life for individuals living with rheumatoid arthritis.

1.5 Impact on Quality of Life

Emotional and Mental Health Effects

Rheumatoid arthritis (RA) permeates far beyond physical pain; its relentless grip extends to the emotional and mental realms, often leading to profound effects on an individual's well-being.

Depression and Anxiety

One of the most prevalent emotional repercussions of RA is the onset of depression and anxiety. The incessant pain, coupled with the uncertainty of the condition, can carve a path toward these mental health challenges. The constant battle against physical discomfort breeds a sense of helplessness, triggering feelings of despair and isolation. Anxiety often takes root due to the unpredictability of flare-ups and the impact they have on daily life. The persistent fear of worsening symptoms or disability perpetuates a cycle of worry and apprehension.

Coping Mechanisms

Despite these challenges, individuals afflicted with RA often develop resilient coping mechanisms. **Acceptance** becomes a pivotal factor—acknowledging the condition and its limitations allows for a shift in focus towards adapting and finding ways to thrive amidst adversity.

Social and Occupational Challenges

Relationships and Work Life

RA's impact on quality of life echoes through social and occupational spheres, straining relationships and work dynamics. The limitations imposed by RA can hinder social interactions, leading to feelings of isolation or even parting from friends and family. The inability to participate in activities or attend events due to pain and fatigue often creates a sense of detachment, impacting the fabric of personal relationships. Similarly, in the professional realm, RA presents formidable hurdles. The unpredictability of flare-ups may disrupt work schedules, leading to absenteeism or reduced productivity. Moreover, physical limitations may necessitate adjustments in job responsibilities or even career paths.

Despite the challenges posed by RA, adopting certain strategies can significantly mitigate its impact on daily life.

The impact of rheumatoid arthritis on an individual's quality of life is multifaceted. Beyond the physical pain, its tendrils reach into emotional well-being, straining mental health, disrupting social connections, and challenging occupational stability. Nevertheless, with a resilient spirit and proactive measures, individuals afflicted with RA can navigate these challenges, fostering a life that, though affected, remains full of purpose and vitality.

2. Foundations of an RA-Friendly Diet

2.2 Essential Nutrients for RA Management

1. Omega-3 Fatty Acids

Sources and Benefits

Omega-3 fatty acids are crucial for managing rheumatoid arthritis due to their anti-inflammatory properties. These fats, primarily found in fish such as **Salmon, Mackerel, and Sardines**, contain eicosapentaenoic acid (EPA) and docosahexaenoic acid (DHA). Both EPA and DHA work to reduce inflammation, easing joint pain and stiffness associated with RA. Research indicates that regular consumption of omega-3s can decrease the production of inflammatory chemicals in the body, potentially mitigating the severity of RA symptoms.

Incorporating Omega-3s into the Diet

Integrating omega-3 fatty acids into your daily diet is relatively simple. Adding fatty fish to meals a few times per week can significantly boost your intake. If fish isn't your preference, alternatives like **Flaxseeds, Chia seeds, and Walnuts are rich plant-based sources** of alpha-linolenic acid (ALA), a precursor to EPA and DHA. Additionally, supplements like fish oil capsules can serve as a convenient way to ensure an adequate omega-3 intake.

2. Antioxidants and Vitamins

Role in Reducing Oxidative Stress

Antioxidants play a pivotal role in mitigating oxidative stress, a process closely linked to the progression of rheumatoid arthritis. Oxidative stress occurs when there's an imbalance between the production of free radicals and the body's ability to neutralize them. This imbalance can lead to damage in joint tissues and exacerbate inflammation, worsening RA symptoms. **Vitamins C, E, and A**, along with **Selenium and Zinc, act as**

potent antioxidants, combating these harmful free radicals and potentially slowing down the disease's progression.

Foods Rich in Antioxidants and Vitamins

Including a variety of colorful fruits and vegetables in your diet is key to obtaining antioxidants and essential vitamins. Berries like blueberries, strawberries, and raspberries are abundant in vitamin C and antioxidants, aiding in reducing inflammation. Additionally, incorporating leafy greens such as spinach and kale provides a rich source of vitamin E, crucial in protecting cells from oxidative damage. Carrots, sweet potatoes, and bell peppers are high in vitamin A, essential for immune function and joint health.

Incorporating omega-3 fatty acids, antioxidants, and vitamins into your diet lays the groundwork for managing rheumatoid arthritis symptoms. These essential nutrients not only help reduce inflammation but also support overall joint health and immune function. By making conscious dietary choices and including a variety of nutrient-rich foods, individuals with RA can potentially alleviate some of the discomfort associated with the condition and support their overall well-being.

2.3 Role of Gut Health in Rheumatoid Arthritis

Rheumatoid Arthritis (RA) is a complex autoimmune disease that affects millions worldwide. While traditionally viewed as a joint-centric condition, emerging research has spotlighted the profound influence of gut health on RA management. Understanding this intricate relationship opens doors to innovative approaches in treating and potentially preventing RA progression. Within this context, the significance of three pillars — probiotics, prebiotics, and a balanced gut microbiome — surfaces as fundamental.

Balanced Gut Microbiome: A Harmonious Ecosystem

The gut microbiome, a diverse community of microorganisms residing in the digestive tract, holds immense sway over immune function and overall health. In the context of RA, an imbalance in the gut microbiota, termed dysbiosis, has been observed in affected individuals. This dysbiosis often correlates with increased inflammation, exacerbating RA symptoms.

1. Probiotics: Cultivating Gut Harmony

Probiotics, commonly referred to as "good bacteria," are live microorganisms that confer health benefits when consumed in adequate amounts. These beneficial bacteria inhabit the gut and play a pivotal role in maintaining a balanced microbial environment. In the realm of RA, studies suggest that specific probiotic strains could alleviate inflammation and modulate the immune response.

Research trials have shown promising results, indicating that certain probiotics can help reduce markers of inflammation in RA patients. Lactobacillus and Bifidobacterium strains have exhibited potential in regulating immune responses, thereby mitigating the severity of RA symptoms. Integrating probiotics into the diet or through supplements holds promise as a complementary approach to conventional RA treatments.Common probiotics: Yogurt, Pickles(fermented), Kimchi, Buttermilk, Coconut or Almond Milk yogurt etc.

2. Prebiotics: Nourishing Gut Warriors

Prebiotics, often less discussed than probiotics, are non-digestible fibers that serve as fuel for the beneficial bacteria residing in the gut. They essentially act as food for probiotics, promoting their growth and activity. Incorporating prebiotic-rich foods such as garlic, onions, bananas, and asparagus can foster a flourishing environment for these beneficial microbes.

Studies exploring the impact of prebiotics on RA are in their infancy but suggest that these dietary components might contribute to rebalancing the gut microbiome. By nurturing the growth of beneficial bacteria, prebiotics could indirectly aid in mitigating inflammation and potentially ameliorate RA symptoms.

Need more Research

However, while the evidence suggests promise, further rigorous research is imperative to elucidate the precise mechanisms and optimize strategies leveraging gut health in RA management. Personalized interventions considering an individual's microbiome profile, dietary habits, and overall health status hold the key to unlocking the full potential of gut-centric approaches in alleviating RA burden.

Though needed more research between Probiotics, Prebiotics & RA management, adding Yogurt or Pickles to your diet isn't that difficult. And if it can provide an improvement in RA management journey, why not we care about our GUT health.

2.4 Importance of Hydration in Managing RA

While medication and lifestyle adjustments play crucial roles in managing RA, the significance of hydration often goes unnoticed. Adequate hydration is fundamental for overall health, but its role in managing RA symptoms is equally noteworthy.

The Role of Hydration in RA

1.Joint Lubrication and Mobility

Hydration is pivotal for maintaining the synovial fluid that lubricates joints. In RA, the immune system attacks the synovium, leading to decreased synovial fluid and increased friction between joints. Proper hydration helps maintain this fluid, potentially easing joint movement and discomfort.

2.Toxin Elimination

Hydration supports kidney function, aiding in the elimination of toxins and waste products. For individuals with RA, this is essential as inflammation produces metabolic waste that needs to be efficiently removed. Ample water intake assists in flushing out these toxins, potentially alleviating the burden on inflamed joints.

3.Reduction of Inflammation

Dehydration can exacerbate inflammation in the body. In RA, inflammation is a major contributor to joint pain and damage. Proper hydration may help reduce overall inflammation, offering some relief from RA symptoms.

How Much Water is Enough?

Individual Needs: There isn't a one-size-fits-all recommendation for water intake. Factors such as age, weight, climate, activity level, and overall health influence the amount of water needed. However, a general guideline is to aim for 8-10 glasses (64-80 ounces) of water daily.

Hydrating Beyond Water

1. **Dietary Sources:** Fruits like watermelon, strawberries, and oranges, as well as vegetables like cucumbers and tomatoes, contain high water content, contributing to overall hydration. Including these in the diet can supplement water intake.

2. **Herbal Teas and Broths:** Herbal teas and clear broths can be additional sources of hydration, especially for those who find it challenging to consume large quantities of water daily.

Tips for Maintaining Hydration with RA

1. **Set Reminders:** Individuals with RA often manage multiple aspects of their health. Setting reminders or using apps can help ensure consistent water intake throughout the day.

2. **Accessible Hydration:** Keep water bottles or hydration stations within easy reach, reducing physical strain for individuals with joint pain or mobility issues.

3. **Balanced Hydration:** While staying hydrated is crucial, overhydration can pose risks. Consulting a healthcare professional to determine an appropriate hydration plan is advisable, especially for those with existing medical conditions.

Hydration is a foundational aspect of managing RA. It plays a multifaceted role, from joint lubrication to toxin elimination and inflammation reduction. Integrating proper hydration practices into daily routines can significantly contribute to alleviating RA symptoms and improving overall well-being. However, it's vital to tailor hydration strategies to individual needs and seek guidance from healthcare providers for personalized recommendations.

2.6 Meal Planning and Preparation Tips

1. Creating an RA-friendly meal plan

Balancing Nutrients and Variety

An RA-friendly meal plan is the cornerstone of managing rheumatoid arthritis through diet. It's not just about what you eat but also how the nutrients interact to support your body's needs. **Balance is key**. Aim for a variety of nutrients from different sources: lean proteins like fish and poultry, whole grains, colorful fruits and vegetables, and healthy fats from sources like nuts and olive oil.

Meal Prepping for Convenience

For those navigating the challenges of RA, meal prepping can be a game-changer. Spend some time on a day that works for you, prepping ingredients and even whole meals. Chop vegetables, marinate proteins, and portion out grains. This not only saves time during the week but also reduces the physical strain of cooking every day.

2. Cooking Methods and Techniques

Anti-inflammatory Cooking Practices

Cooking methods play a pivotal role in maintaining the anti-inflammatory benefits of foods. Opt for methods like **steaming, baking, or grilling over frying**. Steaming helps retain nutrients without adding excess fats, while baking and grilling can bring out flavors without compromising nutritional value. Avoiding high-heat frying can also help minimize the formation of harmful compounds.

Tips for Easy, Joint-friendly Cooking

RA often affects joint mobility and strength, making certain cooking techniques challenging. Embrace kitchen tools that make tasks easier, like jar openers, ergonomic utensils, or electric appliances such as food processors and slow cookers. These gadgets significantly reduce the strain on your joints while preparing meals. (Crafting RA friendly Kitchen will be discussed in detail in later chapters)

Creating an RA-friendly meal plan involves mindful consideration of nutrients and variety. Balancing proteins, grains, fruits, and vegetables ensures a diverse range of nutrients crucial for managing RA symptoms. Meanwhile, meal prepping can be a boon, saving time and energy throughout the week.

In terms of cooking methods, anti-inflammatory practices such as steaming, baking, or grilling help preserve the nutritional integrity of foods. These methods also mitigate the formation of compounds that could exacerbate inflammation. Additionally, adopting joint-friendly cooking tips and utilizing specialized kitchen tools can significantly reduce strain and discomfort while preparing meals.

Meal planning and preparation, when tailored to accommodate RA challenges, become an integral part of managing symptoms and promoting overall well-being.

seeds ensures a diverse nutrient intake, promoting a robust immune system and aiding in the fight against RA symptoms.

B. Sample Meal Ideas and Recipes

Breakfast

Start the day with a nutrient-packed breakfast that sets a positive tone. Consider a smoothie bowl filled with vibrant berries, spinach for added nutrients, a scoop of plant-based protein powder, and a dollop of Greek yogurt for probiotics. Alternatively, oatmeal topped with nuts, seeds, and diced fruits provides a warm and filling option while offering a blend of essential nutrients.

Lunch

Craft a lunch that continues the trend of inflammation-fighting ingredients. A colorful salad loaded with leafy greens, colorful veggies, grilled chicken or tofu, and a drizzle of olive oil and lemon dressing offers a refreshing and nutrient-rich meal. For a heartier option, opt for a quinoa bowl with roasted vegetables, chickpeas, and a sprinkle of turmeric for its anti-inflammatory properties.

Dinner

Dinner should aim for satiety and nourishment. Consider a grilled salmon fillet paired with roasted sweet potatoes and steamed broccoli—a combination abundant in omega-3s, vitamins, and fiber. Another option could be a stir-fry featuring lean protein, such as tofu or shrimp, with a medley of vegetables and quinoa, seasoned with anti-inflammatory spices like ginger and garlic.

Snacks

Snacks play a role in maintaining energy levels and preventing overindulgence during main meals. Opt for a handful of mixed nuts, a piece of fruit with a serving of Greek yogurt, or veggies with hummus for a satisfying and nutritious snack between meals.

Creating an anti-inflammatory plate isn't just about individual meals; it's about embracing a holistic approach to eating. Consistency in incorporating diverse nutrients, controlling portions, and experimenting with flavorful recipes fosters a sustainable and beneficial dietary pattern for managing RA symptoms. By prioritizing the amalgamation of nutrients and flavors in every meal, individuals can harness the power of food as a tool for RA relief.

3.3 Supplements for RA Support

Supplements and herbs have emerged as adjuncts to managing rheumatoid arthritis (RA), offering potential relief from inflammation and discomfort. Within this landscape, several supplements show promise in reducing inflammation and aiding in the management of RA symptoms.

A. Supplements that aid in inflammation reduction

Turmeric

This vibrant yellow spice contains curcumin, a compound known for its anti-inflammatory properties. Studies suggest that curcumin may inhibit certain inflammatory markers in RA. Dosage guidelines often recommend 500–1000 milligrams of curcumin extract, taken two to three times daily. However, it's essential to consult with a healthcare provider to ensure its safety, especially if taking blood-thinning medications due to its mild blood-thinning effects.

Fish oil

Rich in omega-3 fatty acids, fish oil exhibits anti-inflammatory effects that may benefit those with RA. Research indicates that omega-3s found in fish oil can help reduce joint pain and stiffness. A typical dosage ranges from 1000 to 3000 milligrams of combined EPA and DHA daily. Individuals on blood thinners should consult their healthcare provider before incorporating fish oil due to its potential to increase bleeding risk.

Vitamin D

Often deficient in individuals with RA, vitamin D plays a crucial role in immune regulation. Supplementing with vitamin D may help alleviate inflammation and support overall bone health. Dosage recommendations vary based on individual needs and blood levels, typically ranging from

1000 to 4000 international units (IU) daily. Healthcare providers can determine appropriate dosages through blood tests.

Ginger

This spicy root has been valued for its anti-inflammatory properties for centuries. Ginger contains compounds that inhibit inflammatory pathways, potentially providing relief from RA symptoms. Typically consumed as a tea or added to meals, ginger's dosage can vary. While generally safe, excessive consumption might lead to digestive issues.

Certain studies show anti-inflammatory effect & Swelling of Boswellia on Rheumatoid arthritis. Consult your Physician / Healthcare provider, before considering boswellia.

Consulting with healthcare providers

It is imperative to emphasize the importance of consulting healthcare providers before initiating any supplement or herbal regimen, particularly for individuals with RA. These professionals can offer personalized guidance, considering individual health conditions, potential medication interactions, and optimal dosage recommendations.

While supplements and herbs like turmeric, fish oil, ginger, and boswellia exhibit anti-inflammatory properties and show promise in supporting RA management, their efficacy and safety may vary among individuals.

Understanding appropriate dosages and potential interactions is crucial. Healthcare provider consultation remains pivotal in integrating these adjuncts into an RA relief plan, ensuring they complement conventional treatments without causing adverse effects.

3.4 Long-Term Strategies for Sustained Relief

1. Tracking symptoms and dietary changes

Tracking symptoms and dietary changes plays a pivotal role in managing rheumatoid arthritis (RA) through a dietary approach. This practice involves meticulous observation and documentation of how specific foods correlate with the intensity and frequency of RA symptoms. By maintaining a detailed record of food intake alongside symptom fluctuations, individuals can pinpoint potential triggers and identify patterns contributing to flare-ups. This process empowers them to make informed dietary modifications, eliminating or reducing foods that exacerbate symptoms and emphasizing those that alleviate discomfort.

2. Journaling and monitoring progress

Journaling becomes a critical tool in this journey towards relief. Regular entries detailing daily food intake, symptom severity, and any deviations from the established diet provide valuable insights. Not only does this practice facilitate the identification of trigger foods, but it also serves as a means to measure progress. Over time, a well-maintained journal can reveal trends and correlations between dietary changes and symptom management, offering a roadmap towards sustained relief.

3. Adapting the diet over time

The RA relief diet is not static; it evolves as individuals gain a deeper understanding of their body's response to various foods. Adapting the diet over time involves a process of refinement, where individuals incorporate new findings from their tracking and journaling efforts. This iterative approach allows for the gradual elimination of triggers and the introduction of foods that support overall well-being. It's a dynamic process that necessitates flexibility and openness to experimentation, as what works at one phase may need adjustments in another.

4. Adjusting to changing needs and symptoms

As RA is characterized by its unpredictability, the dietary approach must also adapt to the changing needs and symptoms of individuals. This necessitates a proactive attitude, being attuned to the body's signals and promptly adjusting the diet accordingly. For instance, during periods of increased inflammation, a stricter adherence to anti-inflammatory foods might be beneficial. Conversely, during remission or milder symptoms, there might be room to introduce previously eliminated foods cautiously. This continual adjustment ensures that the diet remains aligned with the body's current state, optimizing relief and long-term management.

The journey towards sustained relief from rheumatoid arthritis through dietary strategies is an ongoing process reliant on active engagement and observation. By meticulously tracking symptoms, maintaining a detailed journal, adapting the diet based on newfound insights, and adjusting to changing needs, individuals can navigate the complexities of RA with greater control and achieve enduring relief.

4. Exercise and Movement for RA Management

4.1 Importance of Physical Activity

Exercise plays a pivotal role in managing rheumatoid arthritis (RA), offering a spectrum of benefits crucial for alleviating its symptoms and enhancing overall well-being. Amidst the challenges posed by RA, integrating regular physical activity into daily routines emerges as a cornerstone for improved joint health and mobility.

1. Benefits of exercise for RA

Joint flexibility and mobility

Engaging in physical activity fosters increased joint flexibility and mobility, which are often compromised by RA. Movement exercises, such as gentle stretches or yoga, play a pivotal role in maintaining and enhancing joint flexibility. These activities help in preserving the range of motion in affected joints, mitigating stiffness, and combating the immobilizing effects of RA.

Strengthening muscles around affected joints

Exercise aids in bolstering the muscles surrounding the affected joints, imparting added support and stability. Strengthening exercises, like resistance training or using resistance bands, target specific muscle groups, thus reducing the strain on the joints affected by RA. This fortification of muscles not only helps in protecting the joints but also contributes to improved functionality.

2. Types of exercises recommended for RA

Low-impact activities

Activities that exert minimal stress on the joints are highly recommended for individuals with RA. Swimming, walking, cycling, and water aerobics stand out as excellent low-impact exercises. These activities offer cardiovascular benefits without subjecting the joints to excessive pressure,

Overcoming Exercise Barriers

Dealing with Fatigue and Pain

Fatigue and pain are common challenges faced by individuals with RA. Listening to your body becomes paramount. Begin with shorter, less intense sessions and gradually increase duration and intensity as your body adapts. Prioritize adequate rest between workouts to prevent exacerbating fatigue.

Pain management strategies, such as applying heat or cold packs before and after exercising, can alleviate discomfort. Additionally, consider pain-relieving medications as recommended by your healthcare provider. Remember, pushing through severe pain isn't advisable and might indicate the need for modifications in your routine.

Modifications for Joint Protection

Modifying exercises to protect vulnerable joints is crucial. Opt for low-impact activities that reduce stress on joints while still providing a workout. For instance, swapping high-impact aerobics with swimming or cycling can significantly minimize joint strain.

Utilize adaptive equipment or props like yoga blocks or resistance bands to modify exercises. Adjusting range of motion or opting for isometric exercises instead of high-impact movements can safeguard joints while still engaging muscles effectively.

Developing an exercise routine for managing RA involves customization, professional guidance, and adaptability. It's about finding a balance between challenging yourself and respecting your body's limitations. By creating a tailored plan, collaborating with experts, and making necessary modifications, you pave the way towards improved joint health and overall well-being.

4.3 Daily Movement and Joint Care

1. Incorporating movement into daily life

Joint-friendly activities

Finding ways to incorporate movement into your daily routine is crucial for managing rheumatoid arthritis (RA). While it may seem counterintuitive, staying active can actually help alleviate joint pain and stiffness. Engaging in low-impact exercises, such as swimming, walking, or gentle yoga, can improve joint flexibility and reduce inflammation. These activities put less stress on your joints while still allowing for increased movement.

Ergonomic adjustments at home and work

Making simple ergonomic adjustments at home and work can significantly ease the strain on your joints. Ensuring that your workspace is set up in an ergonomic manner—properly adjusted chair height, ergonomic keyboard and mouse, and adequate wrist support—can alleviate joint pain, especially in the wrists and fingers. At home, using assistive devices like jar openers, long-handled reachers, or ergonomic kitchen tools can reduce the stress on your joints during daily activities.

2. Techniques for managing pain during movement

Warm-up and cool-down routines

Before engaging in any physical activity, incorporating a proper warm-up routine is essential. Gentle stretching exercises or range-of-motion activities help to increase blood flow to the muscles and prepare the joints for movement. After completing your exercise routine, cool-down exercises can gradually bring your heart rate down and prevent muscles from tightening up. These routines play a crucial role in managing pain during and after movement.

Conversely, there might be periods of lower symptom activity, allowing for increased activity. Seizing these moments to engage in slightly more challenging exercises or extend workout durations can be invigorating. However, it's crucial to proceed cautiously and not push beyond your limits, ensuring you don't trigger a flare-up.

3. Flexibility in exercise plans

Having a flexible exercise plan is essential when managing RA:

Develop a repertoire of exercises that cater to different symptom scenarios. This flexibility allows you to switch between activities depending on how your body feels on a given day.

Incorporate a variety of exercises into your routine. This not only prevents monotony but also ensures you can modify your workout without compromising overall fitness. For instance, combining aerobic exercises, strength training, and flexibility exercises provides a well-rounded routine that can be adjusted as needed.

Consistency in exercise can significantly alleviate RA symptoms and improve overall well-being. By setting achievable goals, seeking support, adapting to symptom changes, and maintaining a flexible routine, you can sustain motivation and consistency in your exercise regimen, empowering you to better manage rheumatoid arthritis.

5. Emotional Well-being and Coping Strategies

5.2 Mental Health Techniques for Coping

Rheumatoid arthritis (RA) presents not only physical challenges but also mental and emotional hurdles. The impact of this condition extends beyond the body, often affecting mental health. Coping with RA requires a holistic approach that encompasses stress management, seeking support, and employing various mental health techniques.

1. Stress Management and Relaxation Methods

Breathing Exercises and Meditation

One effective way to manage stress associated with RA is through breathing exercises and meditation. Deep breathing exercises can induce relaxation by calming the nervous system. It involves taking slow, deep breaths, focusing on inhaling and exhaling rhythmically. This technique helps alleviate stress and anxiety levels, promoting a sense of calm amidst the challenges of living with RA.

Additionally, meditation serves as a powerful tool for mental well-being. It involves mindfulness techniques that encourage individuals to focus on the present moment, fostering a sense of inner peace and reducing the impact of stress on both the mind and body. Incorporating meditation into daily routines can significantly contribute to coping with the emotional toll of RA.

Cognitive-Behavioral Strategies

Cognitive-behavioral strategies play a pivotal role in managing the emotional aspects of RA. These techniques focus on identifying negative thought patterns and replacing them with more positive and adaptive ones. By challenging distorted thinking associated with pain and disability, individuals can better cope with the emotional impact of RA.

This approach also involves behavioral interventions, such as activity pacing and goal setting. Learning to break tasks into manageable parts and setting achievable goals can help reduce stress and improve overall well-being. By altering behavior and thoughts, cognitive-behavioral strategies empower individuals to regain a sense of control over their emotional responses to RA.

2. Seeking Support and Building a Support Network

2.1 Family, Friends, and Support Groups

Building a robust support network is essential for individuals grappling with the emotional challenges of RA. Family and friends often play a crucial role in providing emotional support, understanding, and encouragement. Their presence and assistance in day-to-day tasks can alleviate stress and promote a more positive outlook.

Moreover, joining support groups specifically tailored for individuals with RA can be immensely beneficial. These groups offer a platform to connect with others who understand the challenges firsthand, fostering a sense of belonging and empathy. Sharing experiences, tips, and coping strategies within such communities can be empowering and reassuring for individuals navigating the emotional aspects of RA.

Employing stress management techniques like breathing exercises and meditation can aid in calming the mind. Cognitive-behavioral strategies assist in reshaping negative thought patterns, while seeking support from friends, family, and support groups creates a sense of community and understanding. Integrating these techniques into daily life equips individuals with valuable tools to cope with the emotional toll of living with rheumatoid arthritis.

fostering self-compassion involves acknowledging personal limitations without self-criticism. It's about accepting the body's fluctuations and needs without judgment.

RA might pose obstacles, but it also presents opportunities for personal growth and a deeper understanding of self. Cultivating resilience involves recognizing these opportunities, fostering a positive outlook, and embracing self-care practices that support both physical and mental well-being. Through these efforts, individuals can not only manage RA more effectively but also lead fulfilling lives despite its challenges.

6. Navigating Challenges and Flares

6.2 Coping Strategies During Flares

Rheumatoid arthritis (RA) is a condition that, despite management efforts, can still present challenges in the form of flares. These episodes of increased inflammation and pain can disrupt daily life. Coping with flares requires a multifaceted approach that prioritizes self-care, appropriate medical adjustments, and knowing when to seek professional assistance.

1. Self-care during flare-ups

Rest and relaxation techniques

During a flare, allowing the body ample rest is crucial. Implementing relaxation techniques can help manage pain and reduce stress, which can exacerbate symptoms. Simple practices like deep breathing, meditation, or guided imagery can calm the nervous system and provide some relief. Finding a comfortable position, using pillows for support, can alleviate discomfort.

Integrating **heat or cold therapy** can offer localized relief to inflamed joints. Heat pads or warm baths can help soothe stiffness and soreness, while cold packs can reduce swelling and numb painful areas. Experimenting with these techniques and finding what works best for individual comfort is crucial in managing flares effectively.

Medication adjustments as per doctor's guidance

Consulting with a healthcare provider is essential when adjusting medications during a flare. Adhering to prescribed medications while possibly altering dosages, as directed by the doctor, can help control inflammation and pain. Nonsteroidal anti-inflammatory drugs (NSAIDs) or corticosteroids may be adjusted temporarily to manage severe symptoms. However, it's critical to follow medical guidance closely to prevent adverse effects or complications.

2. Seeking medical help when necessary

Knowing when to contact healthcare providers

Understanding when to reach out to healthcare providers is vital for managing flares effectively. Persistent high levels of pain, sudden swelling or redness in joints, and the inability to perform daily activities could indicate a worsening condition. Moreover, if there are concerns about medication side effects or any new symptoms emerging, contacting a healthcare professional promptly is crucial.

Recognizing the signs that necessitate reaching out to healthcare providers is pivotal in managing flares without complications. Persistent or escalating symptoms, such as uncontrolled pain, joint swelling, or limitations in daily activities, warrant immediate attention. Additionally, any concerns about medication side effects or the emergence of new symptoms should prompt communication with healthcare professionals.

Understanding the individual nature of RA flares is crucial; what works during one flare might not be as effective during another. Therefore, maintaining a journal to track triggers, symptom patterns, and the efficacy of coping strategies can provide valuable insights for future flare management. This information can aid healthcare providers in devising personalized approaches to manage and mitigate future episodes effectively.

By incorporating these strategies and maintaining open communication with healthcare providers, individuals can navigate through RA flares with more resilience and control.

6.4 Building Resilience for Flare Management

1. Building a Flare Management Plan

In the realm of rheumatoid arthritis, flare-ups are an unpredictable aspect. However, constructing a well-thought-out plan can alleviate the tumultuous impact of these episodes. The crux lies in preparedness. Creating a toolkit tailored explicitly for handling flare-ups is essential.

Creating a Toolkit for Flare-Ups

This toolkit should encompass a strategic amalgamation of physical aids, medications, and resources for swift relief. Elements like heat or cold packs, assistive devices, prescribed medications, and contact information for healthcare professionals are indispensable. Equally crucial is understanding the individualized nature of triggers. Knowing the cues that precede a flare-up can enable swift action, potentially mitigating its intensity.

2. Emotional Support During Challenging Times

Flare-ups transcend the physical realm, significantly impacting emotional well-being. Managing the emotional toll is as vital as addressing the physical distress.

Coping with Emotional Distress During Flares

Firstly, acknowledge and validate the emotional response to a flare. Accepting and understanding the frustration, anxiety, or sadness that accompanies a flare-up is paramount. Seeking emotional support is not a sign of weakness but a prudent step toward holistic well-being. Cultivating a support network—comprising friends, family, or support groups—can provide solace during challenging times. Sharing experiences and learning coping mechanisms from others can be empowering.

Developing personalized coping strategies is crucial. Engaging in activities that foster relaxation or diversion from pain, such as meditation, gentle exercises, or hobbies, can be remarkably beneficial. These techniques not only serve as distractions but also contribute to emotional resilience.

The management of flare-ups entails a multifaceted approach, intertwining physical and emotional aspects. Understanding the interconnectedness between the two is pivotal for effective management. By assimilating these strategies into daily routines, individuals can fortify their resilience, enabling them to navigate flare-ups with greater confidence and composure.

2. MBSR in conjunction with conventional treatments

Complementary benefits for RA management

MBSR doesn't replace conventional RA treatments but rather complements them. When combined with medications and other therapies, it can enhance overall well-being and alleviate some symptoms.

The practice of mindfulness in MBSR can significantly reduce stress levels, a crucial factor in managing RA. Stress often exacerbates inflammation and pain in RA patients. By cultivating mindfulness, individuals can better manage their stress responses, potentially leading to a reduction in the severity of RA symptoms.

Moreover, MBSR equips individuals with valuable coping mechanisms. The practice encourages a non-reactive stance towards pain, allowing individuals to respond to it more skillfully. This doesn't imply eliminating pain entirely, but rather altering one's relationship with it, minimizing the emotional toll it takes.

Incorporating MBSR into RA management also promotes self-awareness. This heightened awareness helps individuals recognize early signs of stress or tension, empowering them to employ mindfulness techniques proactively. By doing so, they can potentially prevent flare-ups or manage them more effectively when they occur.

Furthermore, the benefits of MBSR extend beyond symptom management. Studies suggest that mindfulness practices enhance overall psychological well-being. For individuals grappling with a chronic condition like RA, this emotional resilience can be particularly valuable in maintaining a positive outlook and improving quality of life.

7.2 Balancing Work, Rest, and Leisure

Achieving a harmonious balance between work, rest, and leisure is essential in managing RA. It involves a mindful integration of activities that promote physical well-being alongside periods of rest to recharge and heal.

Work demands adjustments that accommodate the condition without hindering productivity. This might include restructuring schedules to allow for breaks or adjusting tasks to minimize prolonged periods of joint strain. Implementing ergonomic practices and tools at work ensures that productivity isn't compromised by RA's challenges.

Rest is equally vital. Prioritizing sufficient sleep and incorporating relaxation techniques, such as meditation or gentle yoga, into daily routines aids in managing pain and reducing stress, both of which can exacerbate RA symptoms. Rest is not just about physical repose but also about mental rejuvenation, offering a respite from the complexities of living with a chronic condition.

Leisure: Balancing work and rest lay the groundwork for the integration of leisure activities, which play a pivotal role in holistic wellness. Engaging in low-impact exercises, such as swimming, fosters joint flexibility and strengthens muscles without exacerbating RA symptoms. Creative pursuits like painting, writing, or gardening not only provide joy but also serve as therapeutic outlets, contributing to mental well-being.

Embracing these holistic lifestyle changes isn't merely about adapting; it's about reclaiming control and enhancing one's quality of life despite the challenges posed by RA. By curating environments that support movement and integrating activities that promote physical and mental well-being, individuals with RA can empower themselves to lead fulfilling lives.

Proper Lighting: Ensure bright, well-distributed lighting to avoid straining eyes and aid in clear visibility.

Fire Safety: Install smoke detectors and consider automatic shut-off features on appliances as a safety measure.

Technology and Smart Kitchen Solutions

Voice-Activated Devices: Utilize voice-controlled assistants to manage timers, set reminders, and control appliances.

Smart Appliances: Explore smart refrigerators or ovens with remote control capabilities for added convenience.

Apps for Organization: Use apps for meal planning, grocery lists, and kitchen inventory management.

Designing your Home & Workspace

Similarly, ergonomic furniture, like chairs and beds designed to provide adequate support, lessens pressure on joints while promoting better posture.

Workspace adjustments are equally crucial. An RA-friendly workspace entails investing in adjustable desks or chairs, allowing for personalized settings that accommodate varying levels of comfort throughout the day.

Crafting an RA-friendly Home & workspace involves a thoughtful combination of accessible design, adaptive tools, strategic planning, and technological aids to create a space that eases the challenges posed by Rheumatoid Arthritis.

8. Managing Medications and Treatment Plans

8.2 Working with Healthcare Providers

1. Effective Communication with Doctors

Effective communication with your healthcare provider is pivotal when managing rheumatoid arthritis (RA). It's not just about conveying your symptoms but fostering a collaborative dialogue that aids in your treatment journey. Asking questions and seeking clarity should become second nature. Don't shy away from discussing uncertainties or seeking elaboration on medical jargon. This clarity empowers you to understand the intricacies of your condition and treatment options.

Asking Questions and Seeking Clarity

When facing a complex condition like RA, asking questions is a fundamental step toward understanding your treatment plan. Start by jotting down queries before appointments. This proactive approach ensures that pertinent concerns aren't overlooked during consultations. From medication side effects to potential lifestyle adjustments, no question is too small. Remember, clarity in understanding your treatment regimen equips you to actively participate in your health management.

Collaborating on Treatment Plans

Your healthcare provider isn't just an advisor but a collaborator in your journey towards RA management. Engage in an open discussion about your preferences, concerns, and treatment goals. Collaborating on treatment plans allows you to align your choices with medical recommendations, ensuring a tailored approach that suits your lifestyle and preferences. A shared decision-making process fosters a sense of ownership over your health, fostering a more positive outlook on managing RA.

2. Importance of Regular Check-ups and Monitoring

Regular check-ups form the backbone of effective RA management. These appointments serve as crucial milestones in tracking your progress and ensuring that your treatment plan is yielding the desired results. Moreover, they offer an opportunity for your healthcare provider to make necessary adjustments to optimize your treatment.

Tracking Progress and Adjusting Treatments

Monitoring your RA progress goes beyond mere symptom tracking; it involves assessing the effectiveness of prescribed treatments. Through regular check-ups, your healthcare provider can gauge how your body responds to medications, spot any potential side effects, and fine-tune your treatment plan accordingly. This iterative process ensures that you receive the most effective and suitable interventions, maximizing your quality of life while managing RA.

Working closely with healthcare providers isn't a passive role; it's an active partnership. By actively participating in discussions, asking questions, and staying engaged in your treatment plan, you become an integral part of your RA management. Remember, your voice matters in this journey, and effective collaboration with your healthcare team significantly influences your overall well-being while dealing with rheumatoid arthritis.

9. The Role of Support Systems

9.1 Family and Caregiver Support

1. Understanding the Impact of RA on Family Dynamics

Rheumatoid arthritis (RA) is not merely an individual's ailment; its impact reverberates within the core of familial dynamics. The onset of this chronic condition often initiates a paradigm shift in family roles and responsibilities. Once mundane tasks may become arduous, altering the equilibrium within the household. The emotional toll of witnessing a loved one navigate pain and limitations can reshape relationships, potentially leading to an amalgamation of empathy and frustration.

RA doesn't confine its effects to physical symptoms alone. Its unpredictability can instigate anxiety and stress within the family unit. The flux of flare-ups and remissions destabilizes the expected routine, demanding flexibility and understanding from family members. As roles adapt to accommodate the limitations imposed by RA, a new familial equilibrium strives to find its balance.

2. Communicating Needs and Challenges

Effective communication forms the cornerstone of navigating the complexities that RA introduces into family life. The person with RA, caregivers, and family members must engage in open, empathetic dialogue. Expressing needs and challenges without reservation fosters a supportive environment where concerns are acknowledged and addressed.

For the individual with RA, articulating limitations, pain thresholds, and the evolving nature of symptoms is pivotal. Clear, concise communication assists caregivers and family members in understanding the fluctuating needs of their loved one. Equally, caregivers should openly convey their own experiences, acknowledging the emotional and physical strains they might encounter while providing support.

Understanding doesn't solely entail verbal communication; non-verbal cues often play a significant role. Observing changes in mood, physical media groups, and specialized platforms provide a virtual haven where members share experiences, seek advice, and extend empathy across borders.

Sharing Experiences and Coping Strategies

The heart of these support groups lies in the sharing of experiences and coping strategies. Within these forums, individuals openly discuss their challenges and victories, creating an ecosystem of mutual support. The collective wisdom of the group often unveils novel approaches to managing RA, from alternative therapies to lifestyle adjustments that prove beneficial.

Members don't merely commiserate; they actively empower each other. The shared anecdotes of navigating the healthcare system, combating fatigue, or coping with the emotional toll of chronic pain become invaluable sources of guidance for those treading similar paths. This exchange, grounded in real experiences, fosters resilience and equips individuals with a diverse toolkit for managing their condition.

Conclusion

In essence, the role of support groups and community resources in the realm of rheumatoid arthritis relief cannot be overstated. They offer a sanctuary where individuals find solace, understanding, and practical guidance.

For those grappling with the realities of RA, seeking out these support systems can be a transformative step. Whether it's a local gathering or an online community, the camaraderie, shared experiences, and wealth of knowledge exchanged within these groups stand as beacons of hope, guiding individuals through the labyrinth of rheumatoid arthritis towards a brighter horizon.

9.3 Professional Support Services

Living with rheumatoid arthritis (RA) involves not just physical adjustments but also significant emotional and psychological challenges. Engaging professional support services becomes imperative in managing the multifaceted aspects of this condition.

Accessing Counseling and Mental Health Services

Seeking counseling and mental health services can be pivotal in navigating the emotional upheavals accompanying RA. The diagnosis often triggers various emotions, from fear and anxiety to frustration and sadness. It's crucial to address these emotions promptly. Professional counselors and therapists can offer tailored strategies to cope with the psychological toll of chronic illness. Their expertise guides individuals to understand and manage stressors, fostering mental resilience to face the daily challenges associated with RA.

Managing Emotional Challenges

RA often intersects with emotional challenges, impacting mental well-being. Dealing with chronic pain, limitations in daily activities, and the uncertainty of the condition's progression can lead to feelings of helplessness and depression. Mental health professionals help reframe perspectives, offering coping mechanisms to deal with these emotions effectively. Through cognitive-behavioral techniques or mindfulness practices, individuals can learn to manage their emotional responses and maintain a positive outlook despite the hurdles imposed by RA.

Working with Occupational Therapists and Specialists

Occupational therapists (OTs) play a pivotal role in enhancing the quality of life for those with RA. These specialists evaluate an individual's abilities and limitations, devising tailored strategies to optimize daily functioning. They offer guidance on adaptive techniques, joint protection, and energy

Being an Active Participant in Treatment Decisions

Your role in managing RA goes beyond following prescribed treatments. Actively participate in treatment decisions by engaging in discussions with healthcare providers. Share your preferences, concerns, and any observations about treatment effectiveness or side effects. Collaboration with your healthcare team is key to tailoring a treatment plan that aligns with your needs and lifestyle. Remember, you are an equal partner in decisions impacting your health.

Empowerment, in the context of RA, is not merely about feeling empowered but actively engaging in actions that enhance control and well-being. It involves taking charge of your health, understanding your rights, seeking information, and advocating for yourself.

Advocacy and empowerment are potent tools in the arsenal against RA. By becoming an advocate for oneself, understanding rights and resources, fostering empowerment through education, and actively participating in treatment decisions, individuals with RA can take proactive steps towards better managing their condition and improving their quality of life.

The journey towards empowerment begins with a single step—recognizing the power within oneself to influence and navigate the challenges posed by rheumatoid arthritis.

10. Sustaining Long-Term Wellness

10.2 Fostering Resilience and Positivity

Living with rheumatoid arthritis (RA) presents a myriad of challenges that can test the limits of one's resilience. Yet, within this intricate web of discomfort and limitations, lies the potential for fostering resilience and nurturing a positive mindset that transcends the boundaries imposed by the condition.

1. Cultivating resilience in the face of RA

Resilience isn't about eradicating the challenges posed by RA but rather about navigating through them with fortitude. It involves acknowledging the reality of living with a chronic condition while actively seeking ways to adapt and thrive despite its presence. This journey begins by reframing the narrative around RA—viewing it not solely as an impediment but as a facet of life that, though impactful, doesn't define one's entirety.

Those who cultivate resilience often embrace a mindset that's flexible, one that doesn't succumb to the trials of RA but learns from them. It involves building a support system, including healthcare professionals, loved ones, and communities that understand and empathize with the struggles. Moreover, embracing self-compassion and understanding that setbacks are part of the journey allows for a more resilient response to the ebb and flow of RA's unpredictability.

2. Positive mindset and coping strategies

Maintaining a positive mindset amidst the challenges of RA is not about ignoring the pain or difficulties but about actively choosing a perspective that fosters hope and strength. This involves adopting coping strategies that help manage the emotional and physical toll of the condition. Techniques like mindfulness, meditation, or engaging in activities that bring joy can significantly impact one's outlook. By focusing on the present moment and finding small moments of pleasure, individuals can alleviate the weight of constant discomfort.

Furthermore, fostering a positive mindset involves reframing negative thoughts into more constructive ones. This shift doesn't negate the difficulties but allows for a different lens through which to approach them. It might involve acknowledging the limitations imposed by RA while also recognizing the strengths and capabilities that persist despite them.

3. Finding joy and fulfillment despite challenges

One of the most potent ways to combat the grip of RA is to actively seek joy and fulfillment. It's about identifying activities, hobbies, or pursuits that bring a sense of purpose and happiness. This might involve adapting hobbies to accommodate physical limitations or discovering new passions that align with the abilities available.

Moreover, finding joy doesn't always necessitate grand gestures; it can stem from small moments of connection, laughter, or simply appreciating the beauty around us. Engaging in meaningful relationships, pursuing creative endeavors, or contributing to causes that resonate can infuse life with a sense of fulfillment that transcends the boundaries set by RA.

4. Embracing life beyond the limitations of RA

Living with RA doesn't equate to being defined solely by its constraints. Embracing life beyond these limitations involves acknowledging the possibilities that exist despite the condition. It's about setting realistic goals and aspirations, understanding personal boundaries, and actively pursuing a life that aligns with one's values and desires.

This might involve seeking out adaptive solutions or accommodations that enable participation in activities previously deemed impossible. It's about asserting agency over one's life and making choices that prioritize well-being while not letting RA dictate the entirety of one's existence.

Summarizing key takeaways from the book

DIET

- Identify and avoid foods that trigger inflammation, such as processed sugars, refined carbohydrates, and saturated fats.
- Incorporate a diet rich in anti-inflammatory foods like fruits, vegetables, fatty fish (with omega-3 fatty acids), nuts, and seeds.
- Consider Probiotics & Prebiotics in diet for your Gut health.
- Supplements like turmeric, ginger, fish oil, and vitamin D play a significant role in managing inflammation and supporting joint health.
- Diversify your meals with a balanced diet.
- Stay well hydrated, it reduces inflammation of your joints.

LIFESTYLE

- Obesity damages your joints more, Reduce your weight to normal.
- Exercises maintains your mobility. Incorporate Aerobics, Swimming, Cycling etc., whichever suits you best.
- Crafting Ergonomic RA friendly Home & Workspace is important to reduce strain on your joints & offer an easier lifestyle.
- Emotional Impact can be managed using Rest, Exercise, Yoga, Meditation.
- Practice Mindfulness – Accept your present.

RA FLARES

- RA flares are crucial moments. Note the details such as triggering foods, duration etc in diary or Apps, so that next flares can be managed accordingly.
- Make a readymade Flare toolkit consists of Medications, heat or cold pads, Physician contact numbers etc.
- Medication Side effects monitoring are crucial & should be immediately informed to your Physician so that necessary adjustments are made.

SUSTAINABILITY

- Lifelong learning should be your goal for effectively managing RA & better lifestyle.
- Develop a Positive mindset to lead a better life than you think.
- Family, Friends, Caregiver plays vital role understanding individuals with RA & offering better support they need.
- Support groups & communities are important in sharing their personalised experiences & any new therapies or treatments available.

WISE DECISION

- Seeking Professional guidance is the wise decision you could make.
- Though this book provides enough guidance to guide you in the right path, you need to consult your Physician & other therapist for the guided & personalised Lifestyle.
- DO NOT TRY any new medications, foods you don't know, new products, therapies promising relief without thorough Research and Consent from your Physician.

Journey Towards Wellness

Congratulations on reaching the final chapter of "The Rheumatoid Arthritis Relief Diet." As you close this book, you're not just concluding a series of chapters but embarking on an empowering journey towards better health and well-being. This chapter is a gentle reminder that the end of this book signifies the beginning of your personal revolution—a journey of self-discovery, resilience, and newfound confidence.

Embracing Change

Change can be daunting, especially when it involves altering habits deeply ingrained in our daily lives. But remember, **every great journey starts with a single step.** Embrace change with an open heart and a mindset focused on progress rather than perfection. This journey is yours, and each step you take towards wellness is a testament to your resilience and determination.

Confidence Through Knowledge

Knowledge is a powerful tool. You've equipped yourself with an understanding of how certain foods affect your body and how to make informed choices that support your health goals. Hold onto this knowledge tightly—it's your compass on this journey. Trust in your ability to make educated decisions about your diet and lifestyle, empowering yourself to take charge of your well-being.

Building Resilience

Living with rheumatoid arthritis requires **resilience—a strength that lies within each of us.** There may be days when the journey feels arduous, moments of frustration, or setbacks. But it's important to remember that resilience isn't about never faltering; it's about bouncing back stronger each time. Cultivate resilience by celebrating small victories, seeking support from loved ones, and staying committed to your goals despite challenges.

The Power of Mindfulness

In the chaos of daily life, practicing mindfulness can be transformative. Take moments to appreciate your body's resilience, savor the nourishing foods you consume, and find gratitude in the small joys of progress. Mindfulness isn't just about meditation; it's about being present and kind to yourself throughout this journey.

You Are Not Alone

Remember, you're not alone on this journey. There's an entire community of individuals navigating similar paths, supporting each other, and sharing experiences. Seek support, whether from support groups, online forums, or within your circle of friends and family. Share your victories and setbacks, and draw strength from the collective wisdom and encouragement of others.

A Journey of Possibilities

As you close this book, envision the possibilities ahead. Your wellness journey is an ongoing process, and with each passing day, you're rewriting your story—a story of resilience, courage, and empowerment. Embrace this journey with optimism and determination. ***You have the power to shape your future and live a life where rheumatoid arthritis doesn't define your limits but rather serves as a catalyst for your strength.***

Your Next Steps

The final chapter isn't an endpoint; it's a springboard to continued growth and progress. Use the tools and knowledge gained from this book as a foundation. Consult with healthcare professionals, explore further resources, and continue to fine-tune your approach to better health.

Remember, this is your journey. Embrace it, cherish it, and let it be a testament to your unwavering spirit. You have the power to thrive despite the challenges, and with each step, you're creating a healthier, more vibrant future for yourself.

Keep moving forward with confidence, resilience, and the unwavering belief that you're capable of achieving remarkable wellness.

You are Brave, Strong, Confident, Beautiful Human Being that Rheumatoid arthritis is just a small obstacle in your journey. It's like traffic slowing down our journey, at the end we reach our destination, no matter what. World is big, Life is short. Enjoy your Life to the Fullest.

Wishing you Strength and Success on your Journey,

Dr. PRITHVI INDIRAKUMAR MANGUDIMARUTHAN

I would love to hear from you.

Send your Feedback, Comments, Story of your Journey, any Queries, anything you want to share with me (drprithvidental@gmail.com)

DIET FOR ENHANCING LIFE

Series of Books by Dr. Prithvi Indirakumar

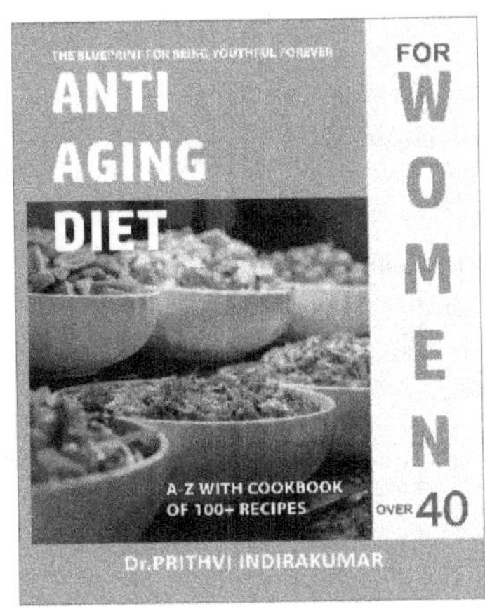

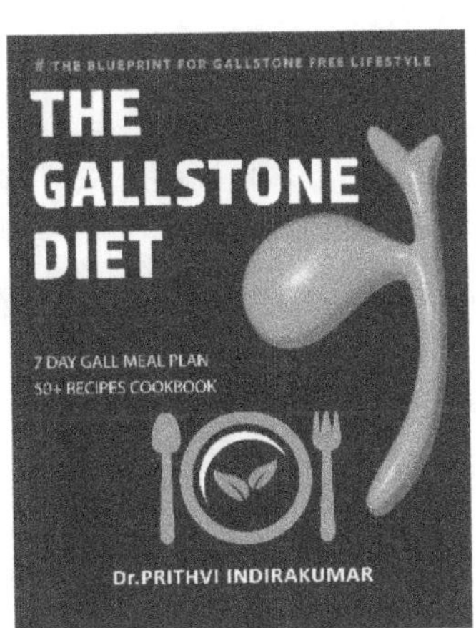

Anti-aging diet for women over 40: A-Z with cookbook of 150+ recipes

The Gallstone Diet: 7-Day Gall Meal Plan with Cookbook of 50+ recipes

- Only Blueprint to provide you longevity
- This book is suitable for **adults both men and women over 40** to have disease free lifestyle through diet which also guides you for the longer healthy lifespan.
- Provides you with a practical approach to start with a **4-week Anti-aging diet plan.**
- Provides you with **150+ recipes for anti-aging life style** to start with.

Only Book you must have to prolong your life just by easy smart diet.

- Get a **detailed diet for Gallbladder health**,gallstone prevention, diet during & after gallbladder removal.
- Also get a detailed knowledge on anatomy & functions of gall bladder.
- Know **A-Z of gallstones**.
- Get a **7- day meal planning** for gallstone diet.
- Provides **50+ gall friendly recipes** for you to start right now.
- **Finest book you ever get on gall bladder health & gall stones**, easier to understand & implement diet for gallstone.